I0455746

Survival:

15 Useful Tips How To Disappear Without A Trace

Table of content

Introduction: Just Another Day... Just Another Footprint

For most of us, as we go about our day browsing the web or swiping our credit cards at stores for purchases, we don't give it much of a second thought. We hardly stop to think of the digital profile that all of these activities are creating. In the grand scheme of things there are two main categories when it comes to the digital footprints that we leave behind. And these two main categories are "active digital footprints" and "passive digital footprints".

When thinking of active digital footprints, think of your Face Book page, because these are online digital billboards where we are actively advertising intimate details of our lives. You post it and the whole world knows about it; pretty simple right? But when it comes to the passive digital footprint that we leave behind without even knowing it—things get considerably more complicated.

This is due to the fact that our passive digital footprints can be stored in an infinitely vast assortment of online environs. To show you just how easy it is to build up your passive digital database, just take a moment to consider all of the links and web pages that you absentmindedly click on any given day. No matter where you are, no matter what device you are using as an interface, every time you make that click, you are dropping off snippets of your passive digital footprint.

Each individual click is known as a "hit" which can be used to track the users IP address, right along with when the site was visited and even what type of computer and internet platform was used to access the site. Active digital footprints need to be managed, minimized, and if you so desire erased completely from public knowledge. In the modern world of rampant identity theft, protecting our most personal of data has become a full time responsibility.

But it's not just your digital footprint you have to worry about either; you also have to be cognizant of your offline tracks as well. Because no matter what you are doing you can't be complacent, in order to truly become invisible you have to be vigilant and practice it every single day of your life. Potential threats to your security can come from anywhere.

I'm not trying to spread fear and paranoia by telling you this, but the fact remains, we live in a very unpredictable world. Everything could be just fine one day and then your whole world could be turned upside down the next. In order to protect yourself as much as possible you have to take hold of your own identity and any corresponding information that comes with it.

You need to be able to control all information that leaves your possession, and whether that means shredding your paper documents before they hit the trashcan or using a P.O. Box to keep your address confidential, all of these things need to be maintained on a daily basis; because in the end its just another day and just another footprint you want to avoid.

Chapter 1: Eliminating your Active Digital Footprint

As was touched upon in the introduction of this book, most of us are actively creating our own digital footprint every single day. It could be as simple as posting a video on You Tube or adding a post to Face Book. The possibility for unique expression today is virtually endless, and as we will see in this chapter so are the consequences.

Facebook

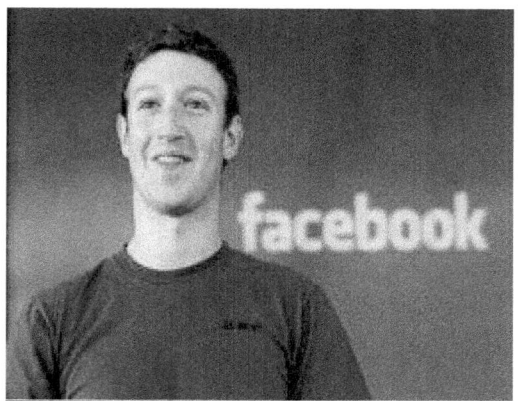

Ever since Mark Zuckerberg broke up with his girlfriend and decided to create a social network for hopeless geeks like himself we have all been at the mercy of this vast digital footprint collector! I am of course being somewhat facetious here but Face Book really is one of the most comprehensive online digital profiles ever conceived of. It is purposefully addictive in nature and pulls more and more information from its users every day they use the platform. It is practically unavoidable.

Even if you are not blatantly posting your address, phone number, and birthday, if you have an active Face Book account there are still no doubt a wide variety of minor details that can be collected about you to form a basic digital footprint. If you wish to minimize the impact of a social media platform like this, always set your Face Book page to private, this will at least prevent you from creating an active digital footprint.

But in the end if you really wish to eliminate your active digital footprint you will need to delete all of your Face Book accounts. Because Face Book itself is a security risk, leaking information on a daily basis, it needs to be controlled. Having that said, the best lesson I could give to someone who is wanting to disappear without a trace. If you have Face Book; get rid of it.

Linkedin

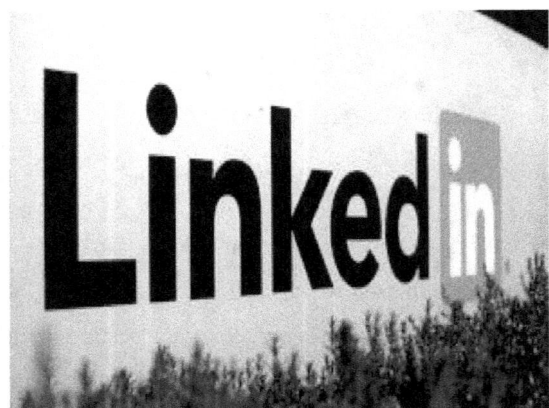

Although Linkedin is supposed to be the premiere site when it comes to meeting professionals and landing the right job, it is also a way to create an immense digital footprint of data that can last for decades. And as it turns out Linkedin is also prime hunting ground for hackers. Because if someone could get a hold of the virtual resume you post on Linkedin they have a veritable treasure trove of information.

Just look at what happened in 2012 when one hacker compromised 6.5 million passwords of registered Linkedin users. These hacks were then followed up by phishing schemes designed to gather even more information from the targets. If you would like to disappear, Linkedin could cause you a major problem. So if you would like to cut down on your digital information you would definitely need to consider getting rid of your Linkedin.

You Tube

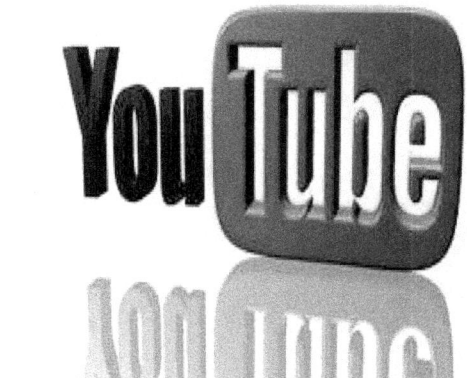

We all love You Tube, we love watching all of the cat video's, music performances, and epic fails that fill our computer. But as entertaining as these things are, our purveyance of them leaves a very unique algorithm in its wake. And much more than this if you have an account and post your own videos through the service you are becoming an active advertising partner. It's not all gloom and doom however, because if you are trying to disappear without a trace it is feasible to use You Tube as a bit of a smoke screen.

You can do this by deliberately posting videos and profile information that has nothing at all to do with you and who you are and then abruptly stop your activity with that account. This could potentially work as diversion for anyone that might be on your trail. So that is my ultimate lesson for you when it comes to You Tube either use it as a disinformation channel for your whereabouts or delete your You Tube account.

Twitter

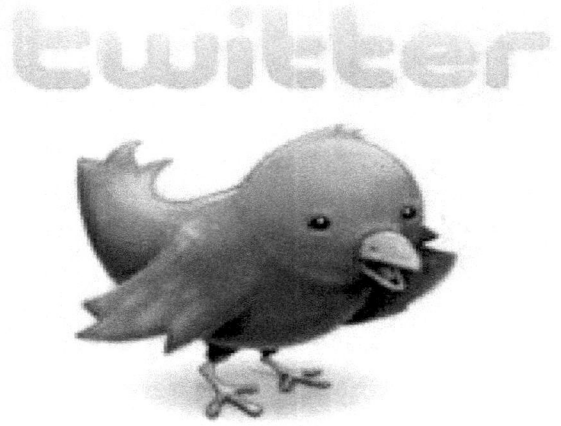

Ah, twitter; the mouthpiece of the world and best friend of Donald Trump! But as much as we enjoy it, whether you are a Presidential candidate or just a regular Joe Schmo down the block, Twitter could be the single most devastating platform when it comes to trying to minimize a digital footprint. Because twitter is like a megaphone announcing to the world your innermost thoughts, and as we have seen during this heated election season, this can be a good thing and a very bad thing!

And one of the toughest things about twitter is that even if you delete posts or even delete your account, anyone who liked your tweets can carry them on for you indefinitely. This can be particularly devastating if your account gets hacked into. I had a friend once who lost control of his account and had someone post ridiculous statements under his name. It took him ages to clear up all the awful things that he never even said!

So let this be a lesson to you; twitter can make and break you. Twitter works as an instantaneous platform to express your own unique persona and if someone were to control this powerful means of expression they will control you. So just to be on the safe side, if you would like to disappear you are going to have to break that twitter habit.

Word press

Word press is great for bloggers and budding writers alike. Being a writer myself, I have lent a few of my own masterpieces to this free writing platform. But all of those opinionated blogs and articles that you cram into word press have a way of sneaking back up on you. They are not going to go anywhere anytime soon, so yes, if you would like to disappear you will have to avoid word press too.

Chapter 2: Eliminating your Passive Digital Footprint

As mentioned in the previous chapter there is a great deal of online activity that we voluntarily contribute to our digital footprint and presence online. But as much as we do things intentionally to build up a digital profile there are many other things that we make constant contributions to that we are blithely unaware of. Because unbeknownst to us there are whole data collecting agencies out there stockpiling all of your absent minded clicks, comments and browsing habits. In this chapter we are going to take a look at some of the most common ways that your passive digital footprints are being created.

Google

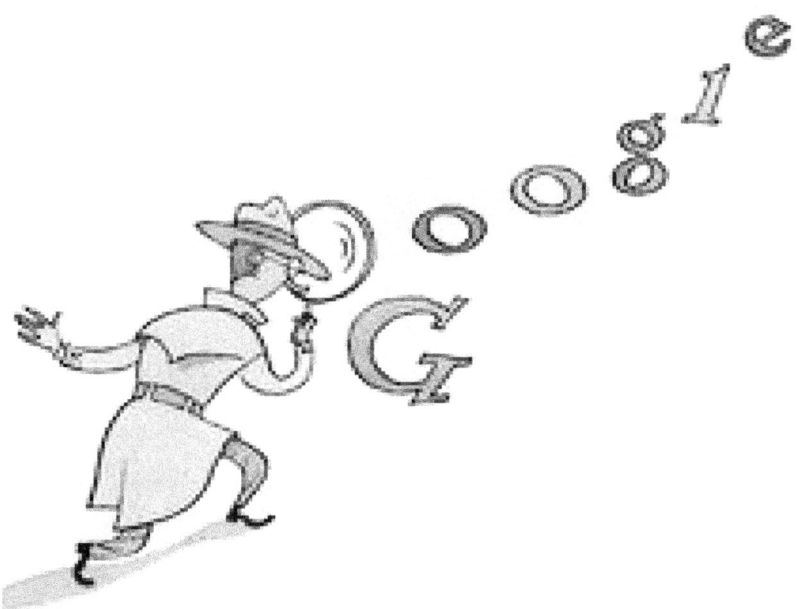

Google is an amazing beast of information and we use it so much that the name has become a part of the lexicon. Surely you have "Googled" something right? The problem is that we all have. And all of this googling by everyone you know has created quite a mountain of information, likes, dislikes and preferences. Like all search engines, Google uses cookies to track where you go while you are on the internet.

These sneaky little cookies gather up all of your personal details so that advertisers can have effective strategies to market products to you based on your online habits. But it isn't only the folks that want to sell you things that keep track of this data. Because there are whole companies known as "Data Gatherers" that store up all the information they can glean from Google and then turn around and sell that info for a price.

From just a thorough scouring of your internet cookies these guys manage to deduce your name, address, age, phone number, previous addresses, occupations and even hobbies. With this passive digital footprint they can follow a trail of cookies all the way back to you. In order to disappear from this digital dragnet you should always optimize your web browser to refuse all cookies.

And not only are the guys at Google busy shaping up these intense digital profiles based upon your clicks and cookies, now because Google is somehow linked to most people's e-mails they are also directly getting information about you through your email account. It is not quite understood why Google wants you to log in with your e-mail in order to search for information on burrito's (or whatever else you are looking up) but it seems to prefer if you are.

The lesson to be learned here is that Google is fast becoming one of the number one data collecting sights on the internet. And so if you really want to disappear you are better off not having this one as a part of your online repertoire. So yes, get rid of Google if you would like to eliminate your passive digital footprint.

Amazon

Amazon is the most popular marketplace on the planet right now and they sell just about everything that you could ever imagine, but did you know that they sell your information as well? Every time you buy something or even just browse through the description of a product Amazon takes note and saves your chosen preferences for a later date. The details of your purchase can be saved for years. Big deal right?

Well—although this may seem rather arbitrary on the surface, these details add up, and can lead to quite an extensive digital footprint. Amazon captures your browsing details by enticing you not only to buy but to comment and rate other products as well. You may think that you are just informing others of how great that last book you read on Amazon was, but you're really just telling them a lot of unnecessary information about yourself. In order to make your online profile vanish, stay away from Amazon.

Ask

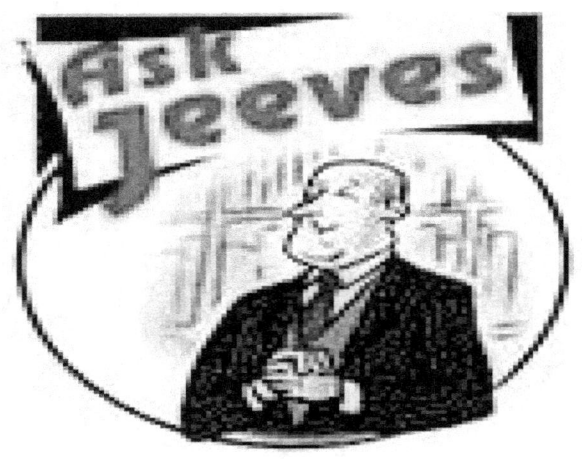

I used to love ask.com. I even remember the good old days when it was known as AskJeeves.com. I loved to see that happy little butler answering all of my questions, and allaying all of my hopes and fears. But I hate to break it to you folks, but that self same company that brought you that chipper butler also took all of your information. Many people have complained about the Ask toolbar that seems to install itself after too many browsing sessions.

This toolbar is unwanted adware at its best and harmful malware at its worst. This software has often been inserted into unsuspecting users computers by bundling together with Java updates. Once installed this toolbar tracks practically everything you do on your computer, storing all of the passive footprints you make for later use. And just like any insidious parasite, the toolbar is not easy to remove. It will fight you all the way, often causing serious system crashes and disruptions just from attempting to delete the program.

To show you just how sneaky the guys over at Ask were when they created this toolbar, they designed it with a delay feature, so that it lays dormant (like a virus maybe?) in your computer and does not present itself immediately after you (accidentally) install it. This toolbar will then show up out of nowhere days later to start sucking up all of your data like a massive cyber leach. So if anything else, in order to avoid this horrible fate, if you are trying to disappear, stay as far away from "Ask" as you possibly can.

E-mail

This lesson in disappearing without a trace is a rather general one, because we all have e-mail. And for most of us, checking our email is as much of a part of our routine as brushing our teeth. But all of this mindless e-mail checking creates quite a trail of passive digital footprints for anyone who might be paying attention, because a simply search of our e-mail log will tell someone where we are when we checked our email, what time of day that we checked and for how long of a duration.

Seemingly simple tidbits of information but when you wish to disappear they can become quite burdensome. The other problem with e-mails is that they can be too easily hacked into. So easy, that even Presidential candidate's such as Hillary Clinton have been hacked. This is because many of us have passwords that are just way too easily guessed. A recent survey found that the most popular passwords for e-mails are 123456, 12345, password, and qwerty.

As you can see none of these are the least bit imaginative, with two of them being just a series of numbers counting forward, one being literally the word "password" and the brilliant "Querty" simply being how the first 5 letters appear on a keyboard, these simplistic passphrases are checked every single day by any resourceful hacker. Even if they don't just guess the generic passwords off the top of their heads, the second they run a hacking oriented computer program all bets are off because that software will skim easy passwords like these right off the top of the list.

And once someone has access to your e-mail they can just about unravel your entire identity, so if you are going to have an e-mail address make sure that it is incredibly complex using a combination of letters, numbers and symbols, and only use it sparingly otherwise you could be compromised. The best way to disappear however is to not have an e-mail address at all. Having that said, I can say that I sympathize completely with Bernie Sanders when he expressed, "I'm sick and tired of hearing about your damn e-mails!"

MapQuest

How many times have we used MapQuest in order to plot our locations when we are lost on some misadventure road trip? In a matter of seconds after plotting in the coordinates you can generate some pretty accurate directions. The only trouble is; directions are not the only thing that MapQuest generates because it also tracks your location and not only that, it stores all of those trips you've ever plotted, leaving all of them stored in the MapQuest database for an indefinite period of time.

Did you enjoy all of those summer trips to Florida? Well guess what? MapQuest enjoyed it too! It enjoyed tracking your whereabouts and traveling preferences during your entire sojourn in the Sunshine State! MapQuest knows exactly where you went because you told them all about it! So if you wish to truly disappear your best bet is to use an old fashioned paper road map!

Chapter 3: Burner Phones, P.O. Boxes and Gerbils Oh My!

So far in this book we have discussed cyber security and how to minimize the shadow that our online habits may create. Now let's take the time to think about all of our offline activities that would need to be minimized and brought under strict monitoring in order to truly disappear from the radar.

Because despite the complexities of today's world, there are still many things you can do to curtail your presence. The main thing to come to grips with is that you are the gatekeeper to your own identity and what it is that gets leaked out. Learn how to control this flow of information and you can control who can see you and who can not.

Cell Phones

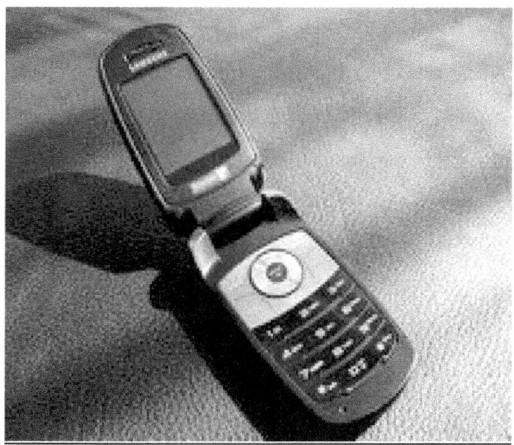

We all love our cell phones, but little do we know that these little gadgets that we all have stuffed right in pockets, purses, and who knows where else are GPS tracking devices. That's right, as long as that phone is turned on, anyone who cares to look into it can find your physical location. Because when your phone is turned on it sends out a constant signal to the nearest cell phone tower, which then gives whoever may be paying attention a pretty good idea of where you are at all times.

So as a rule, if you do use a cell phone, you should turn it off as soon as you are done using it, so you aren't sending out a constant beacon informing others of your whereabouts. This is why having reliable voicemail is important, so you can leave the phone off and then just periodically check it for messages. Only using a phone for when you really need it and turning it off when its not in use is also very conducive for a pay as you go phone or as they are euphemistically referred to "burner phones".

They are named as such because you can basically burn right through these phones and then throw them away. These phones can be used by anyone with none of your personal information attached to it. There is no contract, no deposit, no credit check and no identification required to activate one of these phones. All you have to do is pick one up from Wal-Mart (or wherever you get it from) and pay for the phone and any phone card to supply minutes to the device, all in cash. Follow this lesson and it will be much easier for you to completely disappear when you need to.

Computers

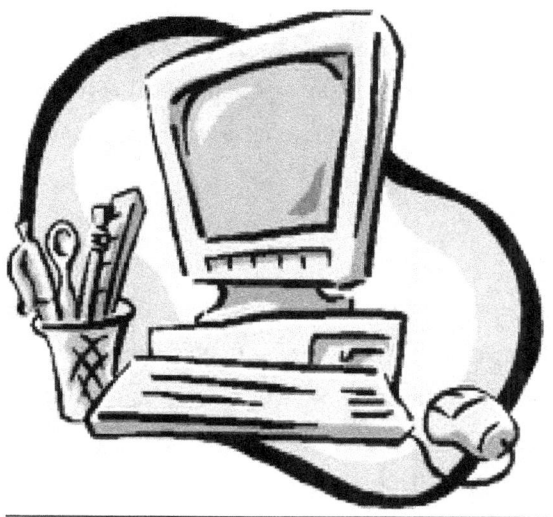

We have been living in the so-called "computer age" for the past 30 years now and you will be hard pressed to found a home anywhere without at least one computing device. Through the internet computer activity can permeate everything we do and we have already touched upon some of the dangers entailed when it comes to online privacy and security. But what you may not realize about computers is that even when they are not connected to the internet they could pose a danger to your personal information.

If anyone breaks into your house and steals your laptop for example, despite the fact that you may have never even took that computer online, your information is now in the hands of thieves. And believe it or not, even without someone physically breaking into your home or hacking into your database through the internet there are still other means by which someone can still your information right off of your computer.

Amazingly if someone had the equipment, they could park a car down the block from your house and pick up your "Van Eck" emissions. This is the steady signal that your computer monitor leaks out and from this signal just about anyone can piece together every single thing on your screen even when you are offline. Sounds pretty scary doesn't it?

Well, as frightening as it is, the only real way to solve these potential breaches in security is to load up our computer with encrypted files. By encrypting your files you are basically jumbling up the main components of the data and recording them in an indecipherable code so that if prying eyes are trying to steal your info they will have a hard time understanding the information that they have lifted. You should also consider creating what is known as "multiple rings" of security or defense.

The first layer of defense for your computer is to make sure that the data contained within it is mobile and can be carried with you when you if need be. The easiest way to achieve this is to use laptops and notebooks; otherwise you should make sure that the hard drive in your desktop is easy to pull out, so you can simply take the hard drive with you when you leave. The next layer of your computer security should be securing the room in which you work with your computer.

All of these precautions may seem rather intense, but as we have seen in this book, if you really want to make 100% sure that know one can compromise your data then you need to really go out on a limb and make that extra effort. So having that said, the first step towards making your room a safe zone free from possible infiltration is to keep the computer away from windows, this is to eliminate the chance of surveillance equipment being used to target your computer. Also if you can try to put a steel plate up on the other side of your door or some other kind of reinforcement to block any radiation or signals that might be leaking from your device.

The next way to safeguard your computer is to use multiple hard drives. You should take two hard drives and install the same operating system on each drive. When you are working with sensitive data you should use the same drive for that purpose, and then when you are done you can ten revert back to the identical drive and take the confidential one out with you when you leave. That way if anyone ever stole your computer you wouldn't lose anything important. These few security measures make it a whole lot easier if you need to disappear.

Use A Gerbil as a Living Shredder

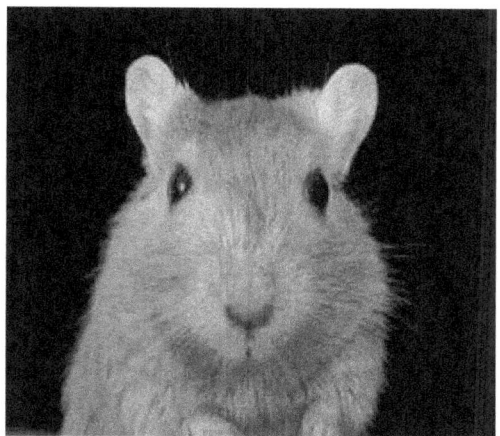

I admit this one sounds awfully strange. And you may have laughed when you saw this heading, but using a Gerbil to shred documents is one of the most effective and efficient means I have discovered when it come to getting rid of sensitive documents. If you have ever had a Gerbil (You know those furry little guys you get from the pet store that look kind of like a cuter version of the rat?) you probably know what I'm talking about though. Because these guys love to shred paper!

They are constantly chewing on stuff and when you hand them strips of paper, they will shred it down into tiny bits and pieces with the consistency of confetti. What I usually do is I take my documents and I shred them through a normal mechanical shredder into conventional strips of shredded paper. But then instead of tossing these shreds into the trash where if someone wanted to they could simply piece them back together again—instead of doing that—I drop the strips right into my Gerbil's cage and he starts working on those pieces of paper immediately.

He's an expert—I've timed the little guy before and he seems to average about one paper strip every 30 seconds. So you give him 8 strips of mechanically shredded paper from one document and he will have all eight of those strips converted into unrecognizable bits and pieces within about 4 minutes. The Gerbil loves this stuff and he will use this now confetti-like paper as his bedding—tunneling in it, sleeping in it, rolling around in it, and yes, even pooping and peeing in it until there is no possible way that anyone could ever glean any possible data from those shredded docs ever again.

I hope you aren't thoroughly disgusted by the concept, but a paper loving animal like a Gerbil can completely annihilate your sensitive documents faster than any mechanical shredder ever could. So yes, for this lesson I seriously suggest investing in a Gerbil just so it can shred all of your documents. Because if you want to disappear and lose your paper trail, a Gerbil's incredible shredding ability is a natural aid in this process.

Post Office Box

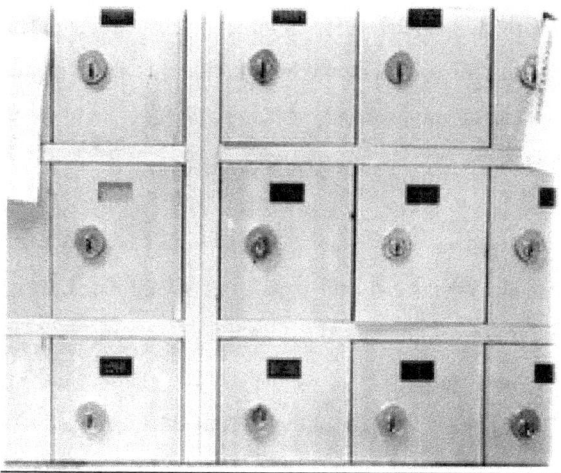

In the information age we think quite a bit about securing our digital information such as e-mails, but we would be very silly to secure our cyber correspondence but then not give any thought whatsoever to our physical mail in the mail box. Because whether you live in an apartment or a house you most likely get flooded with little paper pieces of information everyday and some of it is extremely revealing about your personal assets and situation.

All of this can be solved however by shutting down your fixed mailbox and redirecting all of your physical correspondence to an old fashioned Post Office

Box. The best way to go about doing this is to rent out a private mailbox that is issued by a commercial mail group and then list the P.O. Box under a company name, designating it for magazine subscriptions, or business correspondence.

At the time of opening this P.O. Box your current physical street address is no doubt all over the place, so in order to help that piece of the puzzle disappear, when you move to a new address, do not give it out to anyone and then turn to the P.O. Box that you have already established for all future correspondence. The P.O. Box is not only more secure for your personal information it is also a means to shield your actual street address from prying eyes helping your actual physical location disappear from the radar.

And here's one more tip for helping you shake the paper trail of your old address; get a P.O. Box that is as far away from your starting location as you can. Now I'm not talking about going crazy and renting a P.O. Box in Chicago if you live in New York, but try not to get a P.O. that's in a 5 mile radius of your starting locale. Try to get a P.O. that puts a little bit of distance between you and your starting spot but yet is still convenient enough for you to check at least once a weak.

Limited Liability Company

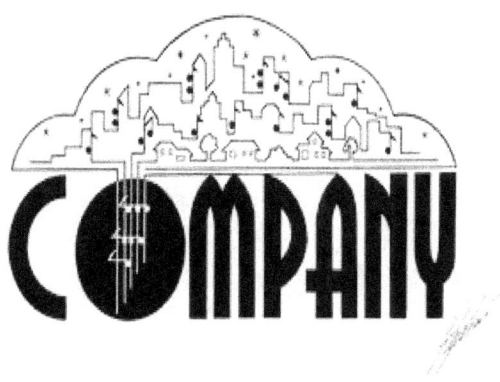

LLC? Surely you have seen this arrangement of these three letters on countless business cards, addresses and solicitation. But what exactly is a Limited Liability Company? Just as the name implies it is a legal entity with very limited liability meaning that no one knows who the owner is unless the owner expressly tells them and it is managed by one single person who lists their LLC as a business address. Obtaining an LLC costs less than $100 and with this you can register cars and license plates under this heading helping you to disappear from unwanted scrutiny.

Conclusion: A Lifetime of Management

We live in a world of constant surveillance. If it's not our online traffic being monitored then it is our physical every day traffic on the streets being scrutinized by thousands of security cameras. Everything in today's world is tracked and compartmentalized inside some database somewhere. So how is it in such a world of scrutiny we could ever hope of holding on to any sense of privacy or security? By common sense and the detailed management of our lives, and I hope that this book has provided you with the tools you need to do just that.

FREE Bonus Reminder

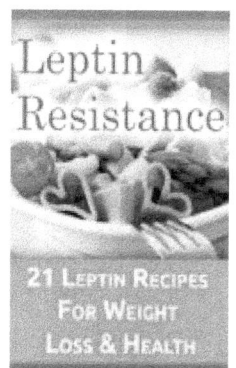

If you have not grabbed it yet, please go ahead and download your special bonus report *"Leptin Resistance. 21 Leptin Recipes For Weight Loss & Healthy Living"*.
Simply Click the Button Below

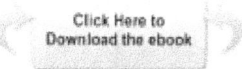

OR **Go to This Page**
http://easyweightlossway.com/free/

BONUS #2: More Free & Discounted Books
Do you want to receive more Free & Discounted Books?
We have a mailing list where we send out our new Books when they go free or with a discount on Kindle. Click on the link below to sign up for Free & Discount Book Promotions.
=> **Sign Up for Free & Discount Book Promotions** <=

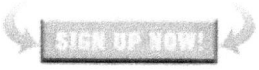

OR Go to this URL
http://zbit.ly/1WBb1Ek